This Gym Tracker Belongs To

____

The human body has 650 muscles.

Date:	Time:
M T W T F S S	

Back ☐	Biceps ☐	Legs ☐	Abs ☐
Chest ☐	Triceps ☐	Calves ☐	Other ☐
Cardio ☐	Forearms ☐	Shoulders ☐	

Exercise	reps	reps	reps	reps	reps	reps
weight						

Exercise	reps	reps	reps	reps	reps	reps
weight						

Exercise	reps	reps	reps	reps	reps	reps
weight						

Exercise	reps	reps	reps	reps	reps	reps
weight						

Exercise	reps	reps	reps	reps	reps	reps
weight						

Exercise	reps	reps	reps	reps	reps	reps
weight						

Exercise	reps	reps	reps	reps	reps	reps
weight						

Exercise	reps	reps	reps	reps	reps	reps
weight						

The only exercise you should hold your breath for is underwater swimming.

Date: | Time:

M | T | W | T | F | S | S

Cardio	Time	Distance	Pace	Interval	Hour	How do you feel after?

Date: | Time:

M | T | W | T | F | S | S

Cardio	Time	Distance	Pace	Interval	Hour	How do you feel after?

Date: | Time:

M | T | W | T | F | S | S

Cardio	Time	Distance	Pace	Interval	Hour	How do you feel after?

Date: | Time:

M | T | W | T | F | S | S

Cardio	Time	Distance	Pace	Interval	Hour	How do you feel after?

Date: | Time:

M | T | W | T | F | S | S

Cardio	Time	Distance	Pace	Interval	Hour	How do you feel after?

Date: | Time:

M | T | W | T | F | S | S

Cardio	Time	Distance	Pace	Interval	Hour	How do you feel after?

The heart is the strongest muscle in the body.

Date:	Time:

M	T	W	T	F	S	S

Back	☐	Biceps	☐	Legs	☐	Abs	☐
Chest	☐	Triceps	☐	Calves	☐	Other	☐
Cardio	☐	Forearms	☐	Shoulders	☐		

Exercise	reps	reps	reps	reps	reps	reps
weight						

Exercise	reps	reps	reps	reps	reps	reps
weight						

Exercise	reps	reps	reps	reps	reps	reps
weight						

Exercise	reps	reps	reps	reps	reps	reps
weight						

Exercise	reps	reps	reps	reps	reps	reps
weight						

Exercise	reps	reps	reps	reps	reps	reps
weight						

Exercise	reps	reps	reps	reps	reps	reps
weight						

Exercise	reps	reps	reps	reps	reps	reps
weight						

Nearly 50% of all young people ages 12-21 are not vigorously active on a daily basis.

Date: Time:

M T W T F S S

Cardio	Time	Distance	Pace	Interval	Hour	How do you feel after?

Date: Time:

M T W T F S S

Cardio	Time	Distance	Pace	Interval	Hour	How do you feel after?

Date: Time:

M T W T F S S

Cardio	Time	Distance	Pace	Interval	Hour	How do you feel after?

Date: Time:

M T W T F S S

Cardio	Time	Distance	Pace	Interval	Hour	How do you feel after?

Date: Time:

M T W T F S S

Cardio	Time	Distance	Pace	Interval	Hour	How do you feel after?

Date: Time:

M T W T F S S

Cardio	Time	Distance	Pace	Interval	Hour	How do you feel after?

For every pound of muscle gained, the body burns 50 extra calories every day.

Date:	Time:

M	T	W	T	F	S	S

Back	☐	Biceps	☐	Legs	☐	Abs	☐
Chest	☐	Triceps	☐	Calves	☐	Other	☐
Cardio	☐	Forearms	☐	Shoulders	☐		

Exercise	reps	reps	reps	reps	reps	reps
weight						

Exercise	reps	reps	reps	reps	reps	reps
weight						

Exercise	reps	reps	reps	reps	reps	reps
weight						

Exercise	reps	reps	reps	reps	reps	reps
weight						

Exercise	reps	reps	reps	reps	reps	reps
weight						

Exercise	reps	reps	reps	reps	reps	reps
weight						

Exercise	reps	reps	reps	reps	reps	reps
weight						

Exercise	reps	reps	reps	reps	reps	reps
weight						

On average, a person walks 70,000 miles in their lifetime.

Date: Time:

M T W T F S S

Cardio	Time	Distance	Pace	Interval	Hour	How do you feel after?

Date: Time:

M T W T F S S

Cardio	Time	Distance	Pace	Interval	Hour	How do you feel after?

Date: Time:

M T W T F S S

Cardio	Time	Distance	Pace	Interval	Hour	How do you feel after?

Date: Time:

M T W T F S S

Cardio	Time	Distance	Pace	Interval	Hour	How do you feel after?

Date: Time:

M T W T F S S

Cardio	Time	Distance	Pace	Interval	Hour	How do you feel after?

Date: Time:

M T W T F S S

Cardio	Time	Distance	Pace	Interval	Hour	How do you feel after?

Exercise makes you feel more energized because it releases endorphins into the blood.

Date:	Time:

M	T	W	T	F	S	S

Back	☐	Biceps	☐	Legs	☐	Abs	☐
Chest	☐	Triceps	☐	Calves	☐	Other	☐
Cardio	☐	Forearms	☐	Shoulders	☐		

Exercise	reps	reps	reps	reps	reps	reps
weight						

Exercise	reps	reps	reps	reps	reps	reps
weight						

Exercise	reps	reps	reps	reps	reps	reps
weight						

Exercise	reps	reps	reps	reps	reps	reps
weight						

Exercise	reps	reps	reps	reps	reps	reps
weight						

Exercise	reps	reps	reps	reps	reps	reps
weight						

Exercise	reps	reps	reps	reps	reps	reps
weight						

Exercise	reps	reps	reps	reps	reps	reps
weight						

Movement in exercise helps relieve stress by producing a relaxation response which serves as a position distraction.

Date: | Time:

M | T | W | T | F | S | S

Cardio	Time	Distance	Pace	Interval	Hour	How do you feel after?

Date: | Time:

M | T | W | T | F | S | S

Cardio	Time	Distance	Pace	Interval	Hour	How do you feel after?

Date: | Time:

M | T | W | T | F | S | S

Cardio	Time	Distance	Pace	Interval	Hour	How do you feel after?

Date: | Time:

M | T | W | T | F | S | S

Cardio	Time	Distance	Pace	Interval	Hour	How do you feel after?

Date: | Time:

M | T | W | T | F | S | S

Cardio	Time	Distance	Pace	Interval	Hour	How do you feel after?

Date: | Time:

M | T | W | T | F | S | S

Cardio	Time	Distance	Pace	Interval	Hour	How do you feel after?

Only 1/3 of adults reach the minimum recommended guidelines for weekly physical activity.

Date:	Time:
M T W T F S S	

Back ☐	Biceps ☐	Legs ☐	Abs ☐
Chest ☐	Triceps ☐	Calves ☐	Other ☐
Cardio ☐	Forearms ☐	Shoulders ☐	

Exercise	reps	reps	reps	reps	reps	reps
weight						

Exercise	reps	reps	reps	reps	reps	reps
weight						

Exercise	reps	reps	reps	reps	reps	reps
weight						

Exercise	reps	reps	reps	reps	reps	reps
weight						

Exercise	reps	reps	reps	reps	reps	reps
weight						

Exercise	reps	reps	reps	reps	reps	reps
weight						

Exercise	reps	reps	reps	reps	reps	reps
weight						

Exercise	reps	reps	reps	reps	reps	reps
weight						

Scheduling rest days helps you meet your fitness goals.

Date: Time:

M T W T F S S

Cardio	Time	Distance	Pace	Interval	Hour	How do you feel after?

Date: Time:

M T W T F S S

Cardio	Time	Distance	Pace	Interval	Hour	How do you feel after?

Date: Time:

M T W T F S S

Cardio	Time	Distance	Pace	Interval	Hour	How do you feel after?

Date: Time:

M T W T F S S

Cardio	Time	Distance	Pace	Interval	Hour	How do you feel after?

Date: Time:

M T W T F S S

Cardio	Time	Distance	Pace	Interval	Hour	How do you feel after?

Date: Time:

M T W T F S S

Cardio	Time	Distance	Pace	Interval	Hour	How do you feel after?

It takes at least 12 weeks of regular exercise to get into shape.

Date: | Time:

M | T | W | T | F | S | S

Back ☐ Biceps ☐ Legs ☐ Abs ☐
Chest ☐ Triceps ☐ Calves ☐ Other ☐
Cardio ☐ Forearms ☐ Shoulders ☐

Exercise	reps	reps	reps	reps	reps	reps
weight						

Exercise	reps	reps	reps	reps	reps	reps
weight						

Exercise	reps	reps	reps	reps	reps	reps
weight						

Exercise	reps	reps	reps	reps	reps	reps
weight						

Exercise	reps	reps	reps	reps	reps	reps
weight						

Exercise	reps	reps	reps	reps	reps	reps
weight						

Exercise	reps	reps	reps	reps	reps	reps
weight						

Exercise	reps	reps	reps	reps	reps	reps
weight						

A pound of muscle burns three times as many calories as a pound of fat.

Date: Time:

M T W T F S S

Cardio	Time	Distance	Pace	Interval	Hour	How do you feel after?

Date: Time:

M T W T F S S

Cardio	Time	Distance	Pace	Interval	Hour	How do you feel after?

Date: Time:

M T W T F S S

Cardio	Time	Distance	Pace	Interval	Hour	How do you feel after?

Date: Time:

M T W T F S S

Cardio	Time	Distance	Pace	Interval	Hour	How do you feel after?

Date: Time:

M T W T F S S

Cardio	Time	Distance	Pace	Interval	Hour	How do you feel after?

Date: Time:

M T W T F S S

Cardio	Time	Distance	Pace	Interval	Hour	How do you feel after?

Switching up your workout will help you lose more weight.

Date:	Time:

M T W T F S S

Back	☐	Biceps	☐	Legs	☐	Abs	☐
Chest	☐	Triceps	☐	Calves	☐	Other	☐
Cardio	☐	Forearms	☐	Shoulders	☐		

Exercise	reps	reps	reps	reps	reps	reps
weight						

Exercise	reps	reps	reps	reps	reps	reps
weight						

Exercise	reps	reps	reps	reps	reps	reps
weight						

Exercise	reps	reps	reps	reps	reps	reps
weight						

Exercise	reps	reps	reps	reps	reps	reps
weight						

Exercise	reps	reps	reps	reps	reps	reps
weight						

Exercise	reps	reps	reps	reps	reps	reps
weight						

Exercise	reps	reps	reps	reps	reps	reps
weight						

Music really does help you work out better.

Date: Time:

M T W T F S S

Cardio	Time	Distance	Pace	Interval	Hour	How do you feel after?

Date: Time:

M T W T F S S

Cardio	Time	Distance	Pace	Interval	Hour	How do you feel after?

Date: Time:

M T W T F S S

Cardio	Time	Distance	Pace	Interval	Hour	How do you feel after?

Date: Time:

M T W T F S S

Cardio	Time	Distance	Pace	Interval	Hour	How do you feel after?

Date: Time:

M T W T F S S

Cardio	Time	Distance	Pace	Interval	Hour	How do you feel after?

Date: Time:

M T W T F S S

Cardio	Time	Distance	Pace	Interval	Hour	How do you feel after?

You're more likely to stick with your exercise plan if you work out with a partner.

Date:	Time:	Back ☐	Biceps ☐	Legs ☐	Abs ☐
M T W T F S S		Chest ☐	Triceps ☐	Calves ☐	Other ☐
		Cardio ☐	Forearms ☐	Shoulders ☐	

Exercise	reps	reps	reps	reps	reps	reps
weight						

Exercise	reps	reps	reps	reps	reps	reps
weight						

Exercise	reps	reps	reps	reps	reps	reps
weight						

Exercise	reps	reps	reps	reps	reps	reps
weight						

Exercise	reps	reps	reps	reps	reps	reps
weight						

Exercise	reps	reps	reps	reps	reps	reps
weight						

Exercise	reps	reps	reps	reps	reps	reps
weight						

Exercise	reps	reps	reps	reps	reps	reps
weight						

Working out can make you better in bed.

Date: | Time:

M | T | W | T | F | S | S

Cardio	Time	Distance	Pace	Interval	Hour	How do you feel after?

Date: | Time:

M | T | W | T | F | S | S

Cardio	Time	Distance	Pace	Interval	Hour	How do you feel after?

Date: | Time:

M | T | W | T | F | S | S

Cardio	Time	Distance	Pace	Interval	Hour	How do you feel after?

Date: | Time:

M | T | W | T | F | S | S

Cardio	Time	Distance	Pace	Interval	Hour	How do you feel after?

Date: | Time:

M | T | W | T | F | S | S

Cardio	Time	Distance	Pace	Interval	Hour	How do you feel after?

Date: | Time:

M | T | W | T | F | S | S

Cardio	Time	Distance	Pace	Interval	Hour	How do you feel after?

Dancing is an excellent form of exercise.

Date:	Time:

M	T	W	T	F	S	S

Back	☐	Biceps	☐	Legs	☐	Abs	☐
Chest	☐	Triceps	☐	Calves	☐	Other	☐
Cardio	☐	Forearms	☐	Shoulders	☐		

Exercise	reps	reps	reps	reps	reps	reps
weight						

Exercise	reps	reps	reps	reps	reps	reps
weight						

Exercise	reps	reps	reps	reps	reps	reps
weight						

Exercise	reps	reps	reps	reps	reps	reps
weight						

Exercise	reps	reps	reps	reps	reps	reps
weight						

Exercise	reps	reps	reps	reps	reps	reps
weight						

Exercise	reps	reps	reps	reps	reps	reps
weight						

Exercise	reps	reps	reps	reps	reps	reps
weight						

Being dehydrated impairs your exercise performance.

Date: | Time:
M T W T F S S

Cardio	Time	Distance	Pace	Interval	Hour	How do you feel after?

Date: | Time:
M T W T F S S

Cardio	Time	Distance	Pace	Interval	Hour	How do you feel after?

Date: | Time:
M T W T F S S

Cardio	Time	Distance	Pace	Interval	Hour	How do you feel after?

Date: | Time:
M T W T F S S

Cardio	Time	Distance	Pace	Interval	Hour	How do you feel after?

Date: | Time:
M T W T F S S

Cardio	Time	Distance	Pace	Interval	Hour	How do you feel after?

Date: | Time:
M T W T F S S

Cardio	Time	Distance	Pace	Interval	Hour	How do you feel after?

It only takes 2.5 hours of moderate physical activity to see cardiovascular benefits.

Date:	Time:

M	T	W	T	F	S	S

Back	☐	Biceps	☐	Legs	☐	Abs	☐
Chest	☐	Triceps	☐	Calves	☐	Other	☐
Cardio	☐	Forearms	☐	Shoulders	☐		

Exercise	reps	reps	reps	reps	reps	reps
weight						

Exercise	reps	reps	reps	reps	reps	reps
weight						

Exercise	reps	reps	reps	reps	reps	reps
weight						

Exercise	reps	reps	reps	reps	reps	reps
weight						

Exercise	reps	reps	reps	reps	reps	reps
weight						

Exercise	reps	reps	reps	reps	reps	reps
weight						

Exercise	reps	reps	reps	reps	reps	reps
weight						

Exercise	reps	reps	reps	reps	reps	reps
weight						

People who don't exercise regularly can lose 80% of their strength by age 65.

Date: Time:

M T W T F S S

Cardio	Time	Distance	Pace	Interval	Hour	How do you feel after?

Date: Time:

M T W T F S S

Cardio	Time	Distance	Pace	Interval	Hour	How do you feel after?

Date: Time:

M T W T F S S

Cardio	Time	Distance	Pace	Interval	Hour	How do you feel after?

Date: Time:

M T W T F S S

Cardio	Time	Distance	Pace	Interval	Hour	How do you feel after?

Date: Time:

M T W T F S S

Cardio	Time	Distance	Pace	Interval	Hour	How do you feel after?

Date: Time:

M T W T F S S

Cardio	Time	Distance	Pace	Interval	Hour	How do you feel after?

Walking briskly burns nearly as many calories as jogging.

Date:	Time:							
M T W T F S S		Back ☐	Biceps ☐	Legs ☐	Abs ☐
		Chest ☐	Triceps ☐	Calves ☐	Other ☐
		Cardio ☐	Forearms ☐	Shoulders ☐	

Exercise	reps	reps	reps	reps	reps	reps
weight						

Exercise	reps	reps	reps	reps	reps	reps
weight						

Exercise	reps	reps	reps	reps	reps	reps
weight						

Exercise	reps	reps	reps	reps	reps	reps
weight						

Exercise	reps	reps	reps	reps	reps	reps
weight						

Exercise	reps	reps	reps	reps	reps	reps
weight						

Exercise	reps	reps	reps	reps	reps	reps
weight						

Exercise	reps	reps	reps	reps	reps	reps
weight						

People who are single work out more than those who are married.

Date: Time:

M T W T F S S

Cardio	Time	Distance	Pace	Interval	Hour	How do you feel after?

Date: Time:

M T W T F S S

Cardio	Time	Distance	Pace	Interval	Hour	How do you feel after?

Date: Time:

M T W T F S S

Cardio	Time	Distance	Pace	Interval	Hour	How do you feel after?

Date: Time:

M T W T F S S

Cardio	Time	Distance	Pace	Interval	Hour	How do you feel after?

Date: Time:

M T W T F S S

Cardio	Time	Distance	Pace	Interval	Hour	How do you feel after?

Date: Time:

M T W T F S S

Cardio	Time	Distance	Pace	Interval	Hour	How do you feel after?

Only 10% of people succeed in losing weight through only dietary changes.

Date:	Time:
M T W T F S S	

Back ☐ Biceps ☐ Legs ☐ Abs ☐
Chest ☐ Triceps ☐ Calves ☐ Other ☐
Cardio ☐ Forearms ☐ Shoulders ☐

Exercise	reps	reps	reps	reps	reps	reps
weight						

Exercise	reps	reps	reps	reps	reps	reps
weight						

Exercise	reps	reps	reps	reps	reps	reps
weight						

Exercise	reps	reps	reps	reps	reps	reps
weight						

Exercise	reps	reps	reps	reps	reps	reps
weight						

Exercise	reps	reps	reps	reps	reps	reps
weight						

Exercise	reps	reps	reps	reps	reps	reps
weight						

Exercise	reps	reps	reps	reps	reps	reps
weight						

People who exercise regularly have higher vitamin D levels in their blood.

Date: | Time:
M T W T F S S

Cardio	Time	Distance	Pace	Interval	Hour	How do you feel after?

Date: | Time:
M T W T F S S

Cardio	Time	Distance	Pace	Interval	Hour	How do you feel after?

Date: | Time:
M T W T F S S

Cardio	Time	Distance	Pace	Interval	Hour	How do you feel after?

Date: | Time:
M T W T F S S

Cardio	Time	Distance	Pace	Interval	Hour	How do you feel after?

Date: | Time:
M T W T F S S

Cardio	Time	Distance	Pace	Interval	Hour	How do you feel after?

Date: | Time:
M T W T F S S

Cardio	Time	Distance	Pace	Interval	Hour	How do you feel after?

Staying active reduces your risk of many cancers.

Date:	Time:
M T W T F S S	

Back ☐	Biceps ☐	Legs ☐	Abs ☐
Chest ☐	Triceps ☐	Calves ☐	Other ☐
Cardio ☐	Forearms ☐	Shoulders ☐	

Exercise	reps	reps	reps	reps	reps	reps
weight						

Exercise	reps	reps	reps	reps	reps	reps
weight						

Exercise	reps	reps	reps	reps	reps	reps
weight						

Exercise	reps	reps	reps	reps	reps	reps
weight						

Exercise	reps	reps	reps	reps	reps	reps
weight						

Exercise	reps	reps	reps	reps	reps	reps
weight						

Exercise	reps	reps	reps	reps	reps	reps
weight						

Exercise	reps	reps	reps	reps	reps	reps
weight						

You're never too old to benefit from exercise.

Date: Time:

M T W T F S S

Cardio	Time	Distance	Pace	Interval	Hour	How do you feel after?

Date: Time:

M T W T F S S

Cardio	Time	Distance	Pace	Interval	Hour	How do you feel after?

Date: Time:

M T W T F S S

Cardio	Time	Distance	Pace	Interval	Hour	How do you feel after?

Date: Time:

M T W T F S S

Cardio	Time	Distance	Pace	Interval	Hour	How do you feel after?

Date: Time:

M T W T F S S

Cardio	Time	Distance	Pace	Interval	Hour	How do you feel after?

Date: Time:

M T W T F S S

Cardio	Time	Distance	Pace	Interval	Hour	How do you feel after?

More than 60% of gym memberships go unused.

Date: | Time:

M T W T F S S

Back ☐	Biceps ☐	Legs ☐	Abs ☐
Chest ☐	Triceps ☐	Calves ☐	Other ☐
Cardio ☐	Forearms ☐	Shoulders ☐	

Exercise	reps	reps	reps	reps	reps	reps
weight						

Exercise	reps	reps	reps	reps	reps	reps
weight						

Exercise	reps	reps	reps	reps	reps	reps
weight						

Exercise	reps	reps	reps	reps	reps	reps
weight						

Exercise	reps	reps	reps	reps	reps	reps
weight						

Exercise	reps	reps	reps	reps	reps	reps
weight						

Exercise	reps	reps	reps	reps	reps	reps
weight						

Exercise	reps	reps	reps	reps	reps	reps
weight						

Half of new gym members quit in their first six months.

Date: Time:

M T W T F S S

Cardio Time Distance Pace Interval Hour How do you feel after?

Date: Time:

M T W T F S S

Cardio Time Distance Pace Interval Hour How do you feel after?

Date: Time:

M T W T F S S

Cardio Time Distance Pace Interval Hour How do you feel after?

Date: Time:

M T W T F S S

Cardio Time Distance Pace Interval Hour How do you feel after?

Date: Time:

M T W T F S S

Cardio Time Distance Pace Interval Hour How do you feel after?

Date: Time:

M T W T F S S

Cardio Time Distance Pace Interval Hour How do you feel after?

Half the people who go to the gym aren't there to work out.

Date:	Time:

M	T	W	T	F	S	S

Back ☐	Biceps ☐	Legs ☐	Abs ☐
Chest ☐	Triceps ☐	Calves ☐	Other ☐
Cardio ☐	Forearms ☐	Shoulders ☐	

Exercise	reps	reps	reps	reps	reps	reps
weight						

Exercise	reps	reps	reps	reps	reps	reps
weight						

Exercise	reps	reps	reps	reps	reps	reps
weight						

Exercise	reps	reps	reps	reps	reps	reps
weight						

Exercise	reps	reps	reps	reps	reps	reps
weight						

Exercise	reps	reps	reps	reps	reps	reps
weight						

Exercise	reps	reps	reps	reps	reps	reps
weight						

Exercise	reps	reps	reps	reps	reps	reps
weight						

In a recent study, 50% of the 2,000 participants said they never even exercise when they're there. Instead, they show up to hang out with friends or check out the opposite sex.

Date: Time:

M T W T F S S

Cardio	Time	Distance	Pace	Interval	Hour	How do you feel after?

Date: Time:

M T W T F S S

Cardio	Time	Distance	Pace	Interval	Hour	How do you feel after?

Date: Time:

M T W T F S S

Cardio	Time	Distance	Pace	Interval	Hour	How do you feel after?

Date: Time:

M T W T F S S

Cardio	Time	Distance	Pace	Interval	Hour	How do you feel after?

Date: Time:

M T W T F S S

Cardio	Time	Distance	Pace	Interval	Hour	How do you feel after?

Date: Time:

M T W T F S S

Cardio	Time	Distance	Pace	Interval	Hour	How do you feel after?

Regular exercise improves your mental health.

Date: Time:

M T W T F S S

Back ☐ Biceps ☐ Legs ☐ Abs ☐
Chest ☐ Triceps ☐ Calves ☐ Other ☐
Cardio ☐ Forearms ☐ Shoulders ☐

Exercise reps reps reps reps reps reps
weight

Exercise reps reps reps reps reps reps
weight

Exercise reps reps reps reps reps reps
weight

Exercise reps reps reps reps reps reps
weight

Exercise reps reps reps reps reps reps
weight

Exercise reps reps reps reps reps reps
weight

Exercise reps reps reps reps reps reps
weight

Exercise reps reps reps reps reps reps
weight

The endorphins released during exercise give you an energy boost.

Date: Time:

M T W T F S S

Cardio | Time | Distance | Pace | Interval | Hour | How do you feel after?

Date: Time:

M T W T F S S

Cardio | Time | Distance | Pace | Interval | Hour | How do you feel after?

Date: Time:

M T W T F S S

Cardio | Time | Distance | Pace | Interval | Hour | How do you feel after?

Date: Time:

M T W T F S S

Cardio | Time | Distance | Pace | Interval | Hour | How do you feel after?

Date: Time:

M T W T F S S

Cardio | Time | Distance | Pace | Interval | Hour | How do you feel after?

Date: Time:

M T W T F S S

Cardio | Time | Distance | Pace | Interval | Hour | How do you feel after?

You're more productive when you're active.

Date:	Time:
M T W T F S S	

Back ☐	Biceps ☐	Legs ☐	Abs ☐
Chest ☐	Triceps ☐	Calves ☐	Other ☐
Cardio ☐	Forearms ☐	Shoulders ☐	

Exercise	reps	reps	reps	reps	reps	reps
weight						

Exercise	reps	reps	reps	reps	reps	reps
weight						

Exercise	reps	reps	reps	reps	reps	reps
weight						

Exercise	reps	reps	reps	reps	reps	reps
weight						

Exercise	reps	reps	reps	reps	reps	reps
weight						

Exercise	reps	reps	reps	reps	reps	reps
weight						

Exercise	reps	reps	reps	reps	reps	reps
weight						

Exercise	reps	reps	reps	reps	reps	reps
weight						

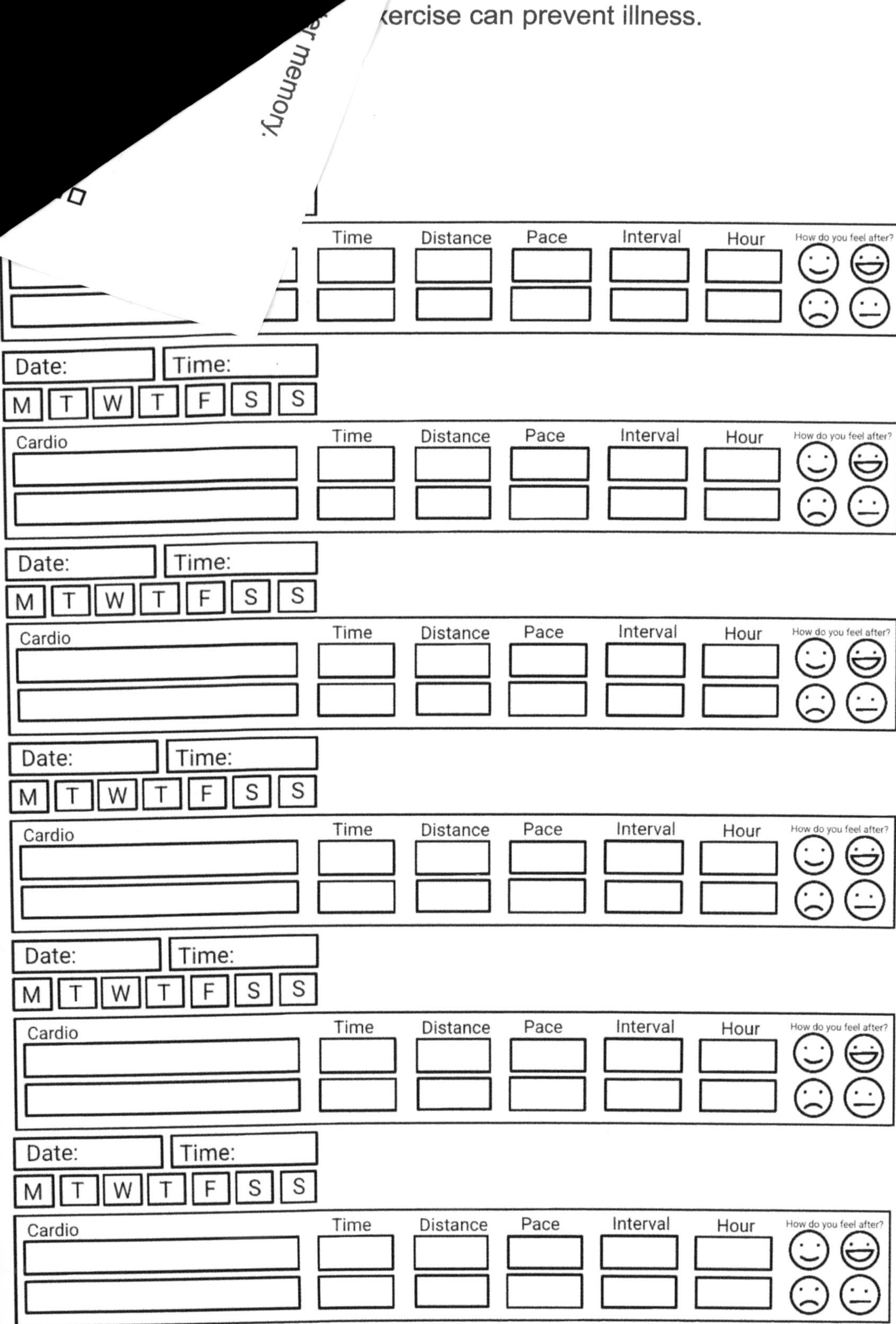

xercise can prevent illness.

r memory.

	Time	Distance	Pace	Interval	Hour	How do you feel after?

Date: Time:

M T W T F S S

Cardio	Time	Distance	Pace	Interval	Hour	How do you feel after?

Date: Time:

M T W T F S S

Cardio	Time	Distance	Pace	Interval	Hour	How do you feel after?

Date: Time:

M T W T F S S

Cardio	Time	Distance	Pace	Interval	Hour	How do you feel after?

Date: Time:

M T W T F S S

Cardio	Time	Distance	Pace	Interval	Hour	How do you feel after?

Date: Time:

M T W T F S S

Cardio	Time	Distance	Pace	Interval	Hour	How do you feel after?

Aerobic exercise is linked to a bett

Date:	Time:

M	T	W	T	F	S	S

Back	☐	Biceps	☐	Legs	☐	Abs	☐
Chest	☐	Triceps	☐	Calves	☐	Other	☐
Cardio	☐	Forearms	☐	Shoulders	☐		

Exercise	reps	reps	reps	reps	reps	reps
weight						

Exercise	reps	reps	reps	reps	reps	reps
weight						

Exercise	reps	reps	reps	reps	reps	reps
weight						

Exercise	reps	reps	reps	reps	reps	reps
weight						

Exercise	reps	reps	reps	reps	reps	reps
weight						

Exercise	reps	reps	reps	reps	reps	reps
weight						

Exercise	reps	reps	reps	reps	reps	reps
weight						

Exercise	reps	reps	reps	reps	reps	reps
weight						

Fat does not turn into muscle when you exercise.

Date: | Time:

M | T | W | T | F | S | S

Cardio	Time	Distance	Pace	Interval	Hour	How do you feel after?

Date: | Time:

M | T | W | T | F | S | S

Cardio	Time	Distance	Pace	Interval	Hour	How do you feel after?

Date: | Time:

M | T | W | T | F | S | S

Cardio	Time	Distance	Pace	Interval	Hour	How do you feel after?

Date: | Time:

M | T | W | T | F | S | S

Cardio	Time	Distance	Pace	Interval	Hour	How do you feel after?

Date: | Time:

M | T | W | T | F | S | S

Cardio	Time	Distance	Pace	Interval	Hour	How do you feel after?

Date: | Time:

M | T | W | T | F | S | S

Cardio	Time	Distance	Pace	Interval	Hour	How do you feel after?

Muscle is built from protein in response to being worked repeatedly.

Date:	Time:

M	T	W	T	F	S	S

Back ☐	Biceps ☐	Legs ☐	Abs ☐
Chest ☐	Triceps ☐	Calves ☐	Other ☐
Cardio ☐	Forearms ☐	Shoulders ☐	

Exercise	reps	reps	reps	reps	reps	reps
weight						

Exercise	reps	reps	reps	reps	reps	reps
weight						

Exercise	reps	reps	reps	reps	reps	reps
weight						

Exercise	reps	reps	reps	reps	reps	reps
weight						

Exercise	reps	reps	reps	reps	reps	reps
weight						

Exercise	reps	reps	reps	reps	reps	reps
weight						

Exercise	reps	reps	reps	reps	reps	reps
weight						

Exercise	reps	reps	reps	reps	reps	reps
weight						

Fat is stored energy, which is broken down and burned when you use more calories than you take in.

Date: | Time:

M | T | W | T | F | S | S

Cardio	Time	Distance	Pace	Interval	Hour	How do you feel after?

Date: | Time:

M | T | W | T | F | S | S

Cardio	Time	Distance	Pace	Interval	Hour	How do you feel after?

Date: | Time:

M | T | W | T | F | S | S

Cardio	Time	Distance	Pace	Interval	Hour	How do you feel after?

Date: | Time:

M | T | W | T | F | S | S

Cardio	Time	Distance	Pace	Interval	Hour	How do you feel after?

Date: | Time:

M | T | W | T | F | S | S

Cardio	Time	Distance	Pace	Interval	Hour	How do you feel after?

Date: | Time:

M | T | W | T | F | S | S

Cardio	Time	Distance	Pace	Interval	Hour	How do you feel after?

Heart rate monitors are not an accurate measure of your workout intensity.

Date: | Time:

M T W T F S S

Back ☐ Biceps ☐ Legs ☐ Abs ☐
Chest ☐ Triceps ☐ Calves ☐ Other ☐
Cardio ☐ Forearms ☐ Shoulders ☐

Exercise	reps	reps	reps	reps	reps	reps
weight						

Exercise	reps	reps	reps	reps	reps	reps
weight						

Exercise	reps	reps	reps	reps	reps	reps
weight						

Exercise	reps	reps	reps	reps	reps	reps
weight						

Exercise	reps	reps	reps	reps	reps	reps
weight						

Exercise	reps	reps	reps	reps	reps	reps
weight						

Exercise	reps	reps	reps	reps	reps	reps
weight						

Exercise	reps	reps	reps	reps	reps	reps
weight						

Ab workouts alone won't give you a six pack.

Date: Time:

M T W T F S S

Cardio	Time	Distance	Pace	Interval	Hour	How do you feel after?

Date: Time:

M T W T F S S

Cardio	Time	Distance	Pace	Interval	Hour	How do you feel after?

Date: Time:

M T W T F S S

Cardio	Time	Distance	Pace	Interval	Hour	How do you feel after?

Date: Time:

M T W T F S S

Cardio	Time	Distance	Pace	Interval	Hour	How do you feel after?

Date: Time:

M T W T F S S

Cardio	Time	Distance	Pace	Interval	Hour	How do you feel after?

Date: Time:

M T W T F S S

Cardio	Time	Distance	Pace	Interval	Hour	How do you feel after?

Crunches and sit-ups do increase your abdominal muscle tone, but you'll never see any abdominal definition if these muscles are covered in a layer of fat.

Date:	Time:

M	T	W	T	F	S	S

Back ☐	Biceps ☐	Legs ☐	Abs ☐
Chest ☐	Triceps ☐	Calves ☐	Other ☐
Cardio ☐	Forearms ☐	Shoulders ☐	

Exercise	reps	reps	reps	reps	reps	reps
weight						

Exercise	reps	reps	reps	reps	reps	reps
weight						

Exercise	reps	reps	reps	reps	reps	reps
weight						

Exercise	reps	reps	reps	reps	reps	reps
weight						

Exercise	reps	reps	reps	reps	reps	reps
weight						

Exercise	reps	reps	reps	reps	reps	reps
weight						

Exercise	reps	reps	reps	reps	reps	reps
weight						

Exercise	reps	reps	reps	reps	reps	reps
weight						

Cardio exercises that burn fat are a key part of building visible muscle tone.

Date: Time:

M T W T F S S

Cardio	Time	Distance	Pace	Interval	Hour	How do you feel after?

Date: Time:

M T W T F S S

Cardio	Time	Distance	Pace	Interval	Hour	How do you feel after?

Date: Time:

M T W T F S S

Cardio	Time	Distance	Pace	Interval	Hour	How do you feel after?

Date: Time:

M T W T F S S

Cardio	Time	Distance	Pace	Interval	Hour	How do you feel after?

Date: Time:

M T W T F S S

Cardio	Time	Distance	Pace	Interval	Hour	How do you feel after?

Date: Time:

M T W T F S S

Cardio	Time	Distance	Pace	Interval	Hour	How do you feel after?

A skinny person isn't necessarily healthier than a larger person.

Date:	Time:
M T W T F S S	

Back ☐	Biceps ☐	Legs ☐	Abs ☐
Chest ☐	Triceps ☐	Calves ☐	Other ☐
Cardio ☐	Forearms ☐	Shoulders ☐	

Exercise	reps	reps	reps	reps	reps	reps
weight						

Exercise	reps	reps	reps	reps	reps	reps
weight						

Exercise	reps	reps	reps	reps	reps	reps
weight						

Exercise	reps	reps	reps	reps	reps	reps
weight						

Exercise	reps	reps	reps	reps	reps	reps
weight						

Exercise	reps	reps	reps	reps	reps	reps
weight						

Exercise	reps	reps	reps	reps	reps	reps
weight						

Exercise	reps	reps	reps	reps	reps	reps
weight						

Working at a computer burns more calories and keeps your metabolism running better than just watching TV.

Date: | Time:

M | T | W | T | F | S | S

Cardio	Time	Distance	Pace	Interval	Hour	How do you feel after?

Date: | Time:

M | T | W | T | F | S | S

Cardio	Time	Distance	Pace	Interval	Hour	How do you feel after?

Date: | Time:

M | T | W | T | F | S | S

Cardio	Time	Distance	Pace	Interval	Hour	How do you feel after?

Date: | Time:

M | T | W | T | F | S | S

Cardio	Time	Distance	Pace	Interval	Hour	How do you feel after?

Date: | Time:

M | T | W | T | F | S | S

Cardio	Time	Distance	Pace	Interval	Hour	How do you feel after?

Date: | Time:

M | T | W | T | F | S | S

Cardio	Time	Distance	Pace	Interval	Hour	How do you feel after?

The pressure on your feet when you run is as much as 4 times your body weight.

Date: | Time:

M | T | W | T | F | S | S

Back ☐	Biceps ☐	Legs ☐	Abs ☐
Chest ☐	Triceps ☐	Calves ☐	Other ☐
Cardio ☐	Forearms ☐	Shoulders ☐	

Exercise	reps	reps	reps	reps	reps	reps
weight						

Exercise	reps	reps	reps	reps	reps	reps
weight						

Exercise	reps	reps	reps	reps	reps	reps
weight						

Exercise	reps	reps	reps	reps	reps	reps
weight						

Exercise	reps	reps	reps	reps	reps	reps
weight						

Exercise	reps	reps	reps	reps	reps	reps
weight						

Exercise	reps	reps	reps	reps	reps	reps
weight						

Exercise	reps	reps	reps	reps	reps	reps
weight						

Every time you take a step, you use about 1/3 of the muscles in your body—and not all of them are in your legs.

Date:	Time:

M	T	W	T	F	S	S

Cardio	Time	Distance	Pace	Interval	Hour	How do you feel after?

Date:	Time:

M	T	W	T	F	S	S

Cardio	Time	Distance	Pace	Interval	Hour	How do you feel after?

Date:	Time:

M	T	W	T	F	S	S

Cardio	Time	Distance	Pace	Interval	Hour	How do you feel after?

Date:	Time:

M	T	W	T	F	S	S

Cardio	Time	Distance	Pace	Interval	Hour	How do you feel after?

Date:	Time:

M	T	W	T	F	S	S

Cardio	Time	Distance	Pace	Interval	Hour	How do you feel after?

Date:	Time:

M	T	W	T	F	S	S

Cardio	Time	Distance	Pace	Interval	Hour	How do you feel after?

Women burn more fat than men during exercise.

Date:	Time:
M T W T F S S	

Back ☐	Biceps ☐	Legs ☐	Abs ☐
Chest ☐	Triceps ☐	Calves ☐	Other ☐
Cardio ☐	Forearms ☐	Shoulders ☐	

Exercise	reps	reps	reps	reps	reps	reps
weight						

Exercise	reps	reps	reps	reps	reps	reps
weight						

Exercise	reps	reps	reps	reps	reps	reps
weight						

Exercise	reps	reps	reps	reps	reps	reps
weight						

Exercise	reps	reps	reps	reps	reps	reps
weight						

Exercise	reps	reps	reps	reps	reps	reps
weight						

Exercise	reps	reps	reps	reps	reps	reps
weight						

Exercise	reps	reps	reps	reps	reps	reps
weight						

Men tend to burn more fat post-workout than women do.

Date: Time:

M T W T F S S

Cardio	Time	Distance	Pace	Interval	Hour	How do you feel after?

Date: Time:

M T W T F S S

Cardio	Time	Distance	Pace	Interval	Hour	How do you feel after?

Date: Time:

M T W T F S S

Cardio	Time	Distance	Pace	Interval	Hour	How do you feel after?

Date: Time:

M T W T F S S

Cardio	Time	Distance	Pace	Interval	Hour	How do you feel after?

Date: Time:

M T W T F S S

Cardio	Time	Distance	Pace	Interval	Hour	How do you feel after?

Date: Time:

M T W T F S S

Cardio	Time	Distance	Pace	Interval	Hour	How do you feel after?

Regular exercise improves your bone density.

Date:	Time:

M T W T F S S

Back	☐	Biceps	☐	Legs	☐	Abs	☐
Chest	☐	Triceps	☐	Calves	☐	Other	☐
Cardio	☐	Forearms	☐	Shoulders	☐		

Exercise	reps	reps	reps	reps	reps	reps
weight						

Exercise	reps	reps	reps	reps	reps	reps
weight						

Exercise	reps	reps	reps	reps	reps	reps
weight						

Exercise	reps	reps	reps	reps	reps	reps
weight						

Exercise	reps	reps	reps	reps	reps	reps
weight						

Exercise	reps	reps	reps	reps	reps	reps
weight						

Exercise	reps	reps	reps	reps	reps	reps
weight						

Exercise	reps	reps	reps	reps	reps	reps
weight						

Both weight-bearing aerobic exercises and strength training exercises can reverse the effects of osteoporosis, reducing the risk of fractures and increasing bone mass.

Date: | Time:
M T W T F S S

Cardio	Time	Distance	Pace	Interval	Hour	How do you feel after?

Date: | Time:
M T W T F S S

Cardio	Time	Distance	Pace	Interval	Hour	How do you feel after?

Date: | Time:
M T W T F S S

Cardio	Time	Distance	Pace	Interval	Hour	How do you feel after?

Date: | Time:
M T W T F S S

Cardio	Time	Distance	Pace	Interval	Hour	How do you feel after?

Date: | Time:
M T W T F S S

Cardio	Time	Distance	Pace	Interval	Hour	How do you feel after?

Date: | Time:
M T W T F S S

Cardio	Time	Distance	Pace	Interval	Hour	How do you feel after?

Cholesterol can give you a more effective work-out.

Date: | Time:

M | T | W | T | F | S | S

Back ☐	Biceps ☐	Legs ☐	Abs ☐
Chest ☐	Triceps ☐	Calves ☐	Other ☐
Cardio ☐	Forearms ☐	Shoulders ☐	

Exercise	reps	reps	reps	reps	reps	reps
weight						

Exercise	reps	reps	reps	reps	reps	reps
weight						

Exercise	reps	reps	reps	reps	reps	reps
weight						

Exercise	reps	reps	reps	reps	reps	reps
weight						

Exercise	reps	reps	reps	reps	reps	reps
weight						

Exercise	reps	reps	reps	reps	reps	reps
weight						

Exercise	reps	reps	reps	reps	reps	reps
weight						

Exercise	reps	reps	reps	reps	reps	reps
weight						

The best time to exercise is 2-3 hours after eating.

Date: Time:

M T W T F S S

Cardio	Time	Distance	Pace	Interval	Hour	How do you feel after?

Date: Time:

M T W T F S S

Cardio	Time	Distance	Pace	Interval	Hour	How do you feel after?

Date: Time:

M T W T F S S

Cardio	Time	Distance	Pace	Interval	Hour	How do you feel after?

Date: Time:

M T W T F S S

Cardio	Time	Distance	Pace	Interval	Hour	How do you feel after?

Date: Time:

M T W T F S S

Cardio	Time	Distance	Pace	Interval	Hour	How do you feel after?

Date: Time:

M T W T F S S

Cardio	Time	Distance	Pace	Interval	Hour	How do you feel after?

Eating protein before your workout increases gains in muscle mass.

Date: | Time:

M | T | W | T | F | S | S

Back ☐ Biceps ☐ Legs ☐ Abs ☐
Chest ☐ Triceps ☐ Calves ☐ Other ☐
Cardio ☐ Forearms ☐ Shoulders ☐

Exercise	reps	reps	reps	reps	reps	reps
weight						

Exercise	reps	reps	reps	reps	reps	reps
weight						

Exercise	reps	reps	reps	reps	reps	reps
weight						

Exercise	reps	reps	reps	reps	reps	reps
weight						

Exercise	reps	reps	reps	reps	reps	reps
weight						

Exercise	reps	reps	reps	reps	reps	reps
weight						

Exercise	reps	reps	reps	reps	reps	reps
weight						

Exercise	reps	reps	reps	reps	reps	reps
weight						

Resistance workouts like weight lifting damage your muscles, and protein is necessary to rebuild them.

Date: Time:

M T W T F S S

Cardio	Time	Distance	Pace	Interval	Hour	How do you feel after?

Date: Time:

M T W T F S S

Cardio	Time	Distance	Pace	Interval	Hour	How do you feel after?

Date: Time:

M T W T F S S

Cardio	Time	Distance	Pace	Interval	Hour	How do you feel after?

Date: Time:

M T W T F S S

Cardio	Time	Distance	Pace	Interval	Hour	How do you feel after?

Date: Time:

M T W T F S S

Cardio	Time	Distance	Pace	Interval	Hour	How do you feel after?

Date: Time:

M T W T F S S

Cardio	Time	Distance	Pace	Interval	Hour	How do you feel after?

About 33% of the average American's calories come from fat.

Date:	Time:

M T W T F S S

Back ☐	Chest ☐	Cardio ☐	Biceps ☐	Triceps ☐	Forearms ☐	Legs ☐	Calves ☐
Shoulders ☐	Abs ☐	Other ☐					

Exercise	reps	reps	reps	reps	reps	reps
weight						

Exercise	reps	reps	reps	reps	reps	reps
weight						

Exercise	reps	reps	reps	reps	reps	reps
weight						

Exercise	reps	reps	reps	reps	reps	reps
weight						

Exercise	reps	reps	reps	reps	reps	reps
weight						

Exercise	reps	reps	reps	reps	reps	reps
weight						

Exercise	reps	reps	reps	reps	reps	reps
weight						

Exercise	reps	reps	reps	reps	reps	reps
weight						

Most people don't need to take vitamins.

Date: Time:

M T W T F S S

Cardio	Time	Distance	Pace	Interval	Hour	How do you feel after?

Date: Time:

M T W T F S S

Cardio	Time	Distance	Pace	Interval	Hour	How do you feel after?

Date: Time:

M T W T F S S

Cardio	Time	Distance	Pace	Interval	Hour	How do you feel after?

Date: Time:

M T W T F S S

Cardio	Time	Distance	Pace	Interval	Hour	How do you feel after?

Date: Time:

M T W T F S S

Cardio	Time	Distance	Pace	Interval	Hour	How do you feel after?

Date: Time:

M T W T F S S

Cardio	Time	Distance	Pace	Interval	Hour	How do you feel after?

Stretching before you run can actually lower your endurance.

Date: | Time:

M T W T F S S

Back ☐ Biceps ☐ Legs ☐ Abs ☐
Chest ☐ Triceps ☐ Calves ☐ Other ☐
Cardio ☐ Forearms ☐ Shoulders ☐

Exercise	reps	reps	reps	reps	reps	reps
weight						

Exercise	reps	reps	reps	reps	reps	reps
weight						

Exercise	reps	reps	reps	reps	reps	reps
weight						

Exercise	reps	reps	reps	reps	reps	reps
weight						

Exercise	reps	reps	reps	reps	reps	reps
weight						

Exercise	reps	reps	reps	reps	reps	reps
weight						

Exercise	reps	reps	reps	reps	reps	reps
weight						

Exercise	reps	reps	reps	reps	reps	reps
weight						

Heavy workouts in the morning can compromise your immune system.

Date: Time:

M T W T F S S

Cardio	Time	Distance	Pace	Interval	Hour	How do you feel after?

Date: Time:

M T W T F S S

Cardio	Time	Distance	Pace	Interval	Hour	How do you feel after?

Date: Time:

M T W T F S S

Cardio	Time	Distance	Pace	Interval	Hour	How do you feel after?

Date: Time:

M T W T F S S

Cardio	Time	Distance	Pace	Interval	Hour	How do you feel after?

Date: Time:

M T W T F S S

Cardio	Time	Distance	Pace	Interval	Hour	How do you feel after?

Date: Time:

M T W T F S S

Cardio	Time	Distance	Pace	Interval	Hour	How do you feel after?

Working out increases your lifespan.

Date: | Time:

M T W T F S S

Back ☐ Biceps ☐ Legs ☐ Abs ☐
Chest ☐ Triceps ☐ Calves ☐ Other ☐
Cardio ☐ Forearms ☐ Shoulders ☐

Exercise	reps	reps	reps	reps	reps	reps
weight						

Exercise	reps	reps	reps	reps	reps	reps
weight						

Exercise	reps	reps	reps	reps	reps	reps
weight						

Exercise	reps	reps	reps	reps	reps	reps
weight						

Exercise	reps	reps	reps	reps	reps	reps
weight						

Exercise	reps	reps	reps	reps	reps	reps
weight						

Exercise	reps	reps	reps	reps	reps	reps
weight						

Exercise	reps	reps	reps	reps	reps	reps
weight						

When you break a sweat, your blood pressure lowers for 16 hours afterwards.

Date: Time:

M T W T F S S

Cardio	Time	Distance	Pace	Interval	Hour	How do you feel after?

Date: Time:

M T W T F S S

Cardio	Time	Distance	Pace	Interval	Hour	How do you feel after?

Date: Time:

M T W T F S S

Cardio	Time	Distance	Pace	Interval	Hour	How do you feel after?

Date: Time:

M T W T F S S

Cardio	Time	Distance	Pace	Interval	Hour	How do you feel after?

Date: Time:

M T W T F S S

Cardio	Time	Distance	Pace	Interval	Hour	How do you feel after?

Date: Time:

M T W T F S S

Cardio	Time	Distance	Pace	Interval	Hour	How do you feel after?

Everyone can reap the benefits of physical activity, regardless of age, shape or size.

Date:	Time:
M T W T F S S	

Back ☐	Biceps ☐	Legs ☐	Abs ☐
Chest ☐	Triceps ☐	Calves ☐	Other ☐
Cardio ☐	Forearms ☐	Shoulders ☐	

Exercise	reps	reps	reps	reps	reps	reps
weight						

Exercise	reps	reps	reps	reps	reps	reps
weight						

Exercise	reps	reps	reps	reps	reps	reps
weight						

Exercise	reps	reps	reps	reps	reps	reps
weight						

Exercise	reps	reps	reps	reps	reps	reps
weight						

Exercise	reps	reps	reps	reps	reps	reps
weight						

Exercise	reps	reps	reps	reps	reps	reps
weight						

Exercise	reps	reps	reps	reps	reps	reps
weight						

Regular physical activity, combined with a healthy diet, can help prevent and manage Type 2 Diabetes.

Date: | Time:

M | T | W | T | F | S | S

Cardio	Time	Distance	Pace	Interval	Hour	How do you feel after?

Date: | Time:

M | T | W | T | F | S | S

Cardio	Time	Distance	Pace	Interval	Hour	How do you feel after?

Date: | Time:

M | T | W | T | F | S | S

Cardio	Time	Distance	Pace	Interval	Hour	How do you feel after?

Date: | Time:

M | T | W | T | F | S | S

Cardio	Time	Distance	Pace	Interval	Hour	How do you feel after?

Date: | Time:

M | T | W | T | F | S | S

Cardio	Time	Distance	Pace	Interval	Hour	How do you feel after?

Date: | Time:

M | T | W | T | F | S | S

Cardio	Time	Distance	Pace	Interval	Hour	How do you feel after?

Regular physical exercise can help you sleep better.

Date:	Time:
M T W T F S S	

Back ☐ Biceps ☐ Legs ☐ Abs ☐
Chest ☐ Triceps ☐ Calves ☐ Other ☐
Cardio ☐ Forearms ☐ Shoulders ☐

Exercise	reps	reps	reps	reps	reps	reps
weight						

Exercise	reps	reps	reps	reps	reps	reps
weight						

Exercise	reps	reps	reps	reps	reps	reps
weight						

Exercise	reps	reps	reps	reps	reps	reps
weight						

Exercise	reps	reps	reps	reps	reps	reps
weight						

Exercise	reps	reps	reps	reps	reps	reps
weight						

Exercise	reps	reps	reps	reps	reps	reps
weight						

Exercise	reps	reps	reps	reps	reps	reps
weight						

Sweat is how your body cools itself down. It doesn't equate to calories burned.

Date: | Time:
M T W T F S S

Cardio	Time	Distance	Pace	Interval	Hour	How do you feel after?

Date: | Time:
M T W T F S S

Cardio	Time	Distance	Pace	Interval	Hour	How do you feel after?

Date: | Time:
M T W T F S S

Cardio	Time	Distance	Pace	Interval	Hour	How do you feel after?

Date: | Time:
M T W T F S S

Cardio	Time	Distance	Pace	Interval	Hour	How do you feel after?

Date: | Time:
M T W T F S S

Cardio	Time	Distance	Pace	Interval	Hour	How do you feel after?

Date: | Time:
M T W T F S S

Cardio	Time	Distance	Pace	Interval	Hour	How do you feel after?

Living with anxiety? Regular exercise can help reduce the symptoms of the condition.

Date: | Time:

M | T | W | T | F | S | S

Back ☐ Biceps ☐ Legs ☐ Abs ☐
Chest ☐ Triceps ☐ Calves ☐ Other ☐
Cardio ☐ Forearms ☐ Shoulders ☐

Exercise	reps	reps	reps	reps	reps	reps
weight						

Exercise	reps	reps	reps	reps	reps	reps
weight						

Exercise	reps	reps	reps	reps	reps	reps
weight						

Exercise	reps	reps	reps	reps	reps	reps
weight						

Exercise	reps	reps	reps	reps	reps	reps
weight						

Exercise	reps	reps	reps	reps	reps	reps
weight						

Exercise	reps	reps	reps	reps	reps	reps
weight						

Exercise	reps	reps	reps	reps	reps	reps
weight						

Pinched for time? Even 10 minutes of exercise will help raise your heart rate and maintain fitness levels.

Date: Time:

M T W T F S S

Cardio	Time	Distance	Pace	Interval	Hour	How do you feel after?

Date: Time:

M T W T F S S

Cardio	Time	Distance	Pace	Interval	Hour	How do you feel after?

Date: Time:

M T W T F S S

Cardio	Time	Distance	Pace	Interval	Hour	How do you feel after?

Date: Time:

M T W T F S S

Cardio	Time	Distance	Pace	Interval	Hour	How do you feel after?

Date: Time:

M T W T F S S

Cardio	Time	Distance	Pace	Interval	Hour	How do you feel after?

Date: Time:

M T W T F S S

Cardio	Time	Distance	Pace	Interval	Hour	How do you feel after?

Walking at a brisk pace can burn almost as many calories as jogging the same distance.

Date:	Time:
M T W T F S S	

Back ☐	Chest ☐	Cardio ☐	Biceps ☐	Triceps ☐	Forearms ☐	Legs ☐	Calves ☐
Shoulders ☐	Abs ☐	Other ☐					

Exercise	reps	reps	reps	reps	reps	reps
weight						

Exercise	reps	reps	reps	reps	reps	reps
weight						

Exercise	reps	reps	reps	reps	reps	reps
weight						

Exercise	reps	reps	reps	reps	reps	reps
weight						

Exercise	reps	reps	reps	reps	reps	reps
weight						

Exercise	reps	reps	reps	reps	reps	reps
weight						

Exercise	reps	reps	reps	reps	reps	reps
weight						

Exercise	reps	reps	reps	reps	reps	reps
weight						

It takes the body six to eight weeks to adapt to an exercise program.

Date: Time:

M T W T F S S

Cardio	Time	Distance	Pace	Interval	Hour	How do you feel after?

Date: Time:

M T W T F S S

Cardio	Time	Distance	Pace	Interval	Hour	How do you feel after?

Date: Time:

M T W T F S S

Cardio	Time	Distance	Pace	Interval	Hour	How do you feel after?

Date: Time:

M T W T F S S

Cardio	Time	Distance	Pace	Interval	Hour	How do you feel after?

Date: Time:

M T W T F S S

Cardio	Time	Distance	Pace	Interval	Hour	How do you feel after?

Date: Time:

M T W T F S S

Cardio	Time	Distance	Pace	Interval	Hour	How do you feel after?

Strength training is simply creating work for your muscles through resistance. This can be done in many ways, including using just your body weight.

Date:	Time:

M	T	W	T	F	S	S

Back	☐	Biceps	☐	Legs	☐	Abs	☐
Chest	☐	Triceps	☐	Calves	☐	Other	☐
Cardio	☐	Forearms	☐	Shoulders	☐		

Exercise	reps	reps	reps	reps	reps	reps
weight						

Exercise	reps	reps	reps	reps	reps	reps
weight						

Exercise	reps	reps	reps	reps	reps	reps
weight						

Exercise	reps	reps	reps	reps	reps	reps
weight						

Exercise	reps	reps	reps	reps	reps	reps
weight						

Exercise	reps	reps	reps	reps	reps	reps
weight						

Exercise	reps	reps	reps	reps	reps	reps
weight						

Exercise	reps	reps	reps	reps	reps	reps
weight						

The 'core' includes any muscles that attach to your pelvis, spine and ribs.

Date: | Time:

M | T | W | T | F | S | S

Cardio	Time	Distance	Pace	Interval	Hour	How do you feel after?

Date: | Time:

M | T | W | T | F | S | S

Cardio	Time	Distance	Pace	Interval	Hour	How do you feel after?

Date: | Time:

M | T | W | T | F | S | S

Cardio	Time	Distance	Pace	Interval	Hour	How do you feel after?

Date: | Time:

M | T | W | T | F | S | S

Cardio	Time	Distance	Pace	Interval	Hour	How do you feel after?

Date: | Time:

M | T | W | T | F | S | S

Cardio	Time	Distance	Pace	Interval	Hour	How do you feel after?

Date: | Time:

M | T | W | T | F | S | S

Cardio	Time	Distance	Pace	Interval	Hour	How do you feel after?

www.ingramcontent.com/pod-product-compliance
Ingram Content Group UK Ltd.
Pitfield, Milton Keynes, MK11 3LW, UK
UKHW021925190726
13853UKWH00002B/848